# DANCE ROUTINE FOR SENIORS OVER 60

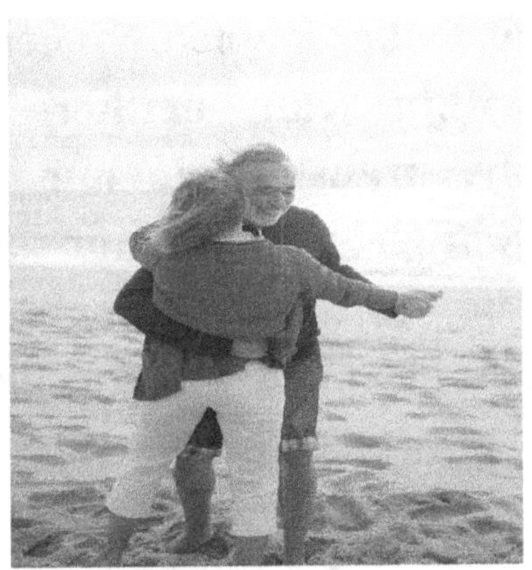

## A Holistic Approach to Aging with Vitality, Balancing Body, Mind, and Spirit for Optimal Well-being and Resilience

### By

### Michelle T. Rills

# Table of contents

# About the Book

A comprehensive guide that transcends the traditional perception of dance as a youthful pursuit. Authored with a deep understanding of the unique needs and considerations of seniors over 60, this book is a thoughtful exploration of the physical, mental, and social benefits that dance can offer to this demographic.

The introductory section sets the stage, providing background on the significance of dance in the lives of seniors and outlining the purpose of the book. It immediately engages the reader, encouraging them to see dance not just as a form of recreation but as a holistic approach to wellness.

Delving into the benefits of dance, the book meticulously explores how it positively impacts physical health, emphasizing cardiovascular benefits, improved flexibility, and enhanced mobility. It doesn't stop there, addressing the profound mental health benefits, such as cognitive function and emotional well-being. The social aspects of dance are given due attention, highlighting how it fosters community, friendship, and a sense of belonging.

Recognizing the unique health considerations for seniors, the book provides a detailed examination of physical limitations and stresses the importance of medical consultation before embarking on a dance routine. It guides readers on choosing appropriate music, incorporating warm-up exercises, and gradually introducing simple dance moves suitable for this demographic.

The book's inclusivity is evident in its exploration of seated dance options, catering to those with mobility challenges. Safety is paramount, with a dedicated section offering practical tips on proper footwear, lighting, and emergency preparedness.

The inclusion of partner and group dances recognizes the social nature of seniors' activities, enhancing the overall experience. Testimonials and success stories peppered throughout the book serve as inspiring anecdotes, illustrating the transformative power of dance in the lives of seniors.

Concluding with a wealth of resources, from online classes to community centers, the book equips readers with the tools to embark on their dance journey confidently. "Dance for Seniors" stands as a beacon, advocating not just for movement but for a joyous, inclusive, and holistic approach to senior well-being through the art of dance.

# Introduction

The golden years deserve to shimmer with vitality, and what better way to achieve this than through the rhythmic embrace of dance? This guide is a compass for seniors over 60, navigating the delightful world of dance routines tailored to enhance physical well-being, cognitive function, and emotional joy. As we embark on this journey, it's crucial to recognize that age should never be a barrier to the sheer enjoyment of movement.

In the opening chapters, we delve into the manifold benefits awaiting those who lace up their dance shoes. From cardiovascular health to cognitive sharpness, the advantages are not merely physical but extend to fostering a profound sense of joy and accomplishment. Safety is paramount, and we discuss the precautions necessary to ensure that dance becomes a source of empowerment rather than a cause for concern.

The guide unfolds progressively, from warm-up exercises designed to gently awaken aging muscles to the intricacies of crafting a personalized dance routine. Whether it's solo footwork or the camaraderie of group dance, we explore how movement can be both therapeutic and socially enriching. Music, a universal language, takes center stage as we discuss its role in motivation and expression.

Throughout these pages, you'll find a roadmap to not only embrace the physical benefits of dance but also to cultivate a community of like-minded individuals. So, let the music play, the body sway, and the spirit dance freely as we embark on a journey that transcends age, proving that the art of movement is timeless and ageless.

# Foreword

In a quaint community nestled among rolling hills, a vibrant transformation was quietly unfolding. Meet Clara, a spirited woman in her sixties who, like many of her peers, found herself at a crossroads of aging gracefully and staying active. One day, inspired by the rhythm of an old tune on the radio, Clara took a leap into the world of dance.

This whimsical journey, mirrored in the pages of "Dance for Seniors: Embracing Wellness through Movement," begins with a melody that transcends the boundaries of time. The introduction opens with Clara's story, narrating the initial skepticism, the nervous laughter, and ultimately, the sheer joy that filled the room as she discovered the rejuvenating power of dance.

The setting unfolds, painting a picture of a community hall that becomes a canvas for diverse stories and experiences. The introduction captures the essence of dance not merely as a physical activity but as a tapestry weaving together social connections, newfound friendships, and a shared sense of purpose among seniors.

As Clara takes her first steps, readers are invited to join her in a dance that defies the stereotypes associated with aging. The pages come alive with anecdotes of laughter, graceful movements, and the collective applause of a community rediscovering the vitality of life through dance.

This story-based introduction not only sets the stage for the practical guidance to come but resonates with the lived experiences of seniors everywhere. As the curtain rises on Clara's dance journey, it beckons readers to turn the page and embark on their own transformative adventure into the world of dance, where the music knows no age and the joy is boundless.

# Chapter 1

## 1.1 Importance of Physical Activity for Seniors

Engaging in regular physical activity is of paramount importance for seniors, as it plays a pivotal role in promoting overall health, vitality, and quality of life during the golden years. As individuals age, there is a natural tendency for muscle mass and bone density to decrease, and joints may become stiffer. Regular physical activity helps counteract these effects, contributing to improved strength, flexibility, and balance.

One of the primary benefits is the positive impact on cardiovascular health. Regular exercise reduces the risk of heart disease, lowers blood pressure, and improves circulation. This, in turn, enhances the efficiency of the heart and lungs, promoting a more robust cardiovascular system.

Physical activity also plays a crucial role in maintaining a healthy weight, which is particularly significant as metabolism tends to slow down with age. By incorporating regular exercise into their routine, seniors can manage weight more effectively and reduce the risk of obesity-related conditions.

Furthermore, engaging in physical activity has profound effects on mental well-being. Exercise stimulates the release of endorphins, the body's natural mood lifters, which can alleviate symptoms of depression and anxiety. Additionally, staying physically active contributes to better cognitive function and a reduced risk of cognitive decline and dementia.

For seniors, the importance of physical activity extends beyond the physical and mental realms—it fosters social connections. Participating in group activities or classes provides opportunities for social interaction, reducing feelings of isolation and promoting a sense of community.

In essence, the significance of physical activity for seniors lies in its multifaceted ability to enhance physical health, mental well-being, and social connections, ultimately contributing to a more fulfilling and active lifestyle in the later years.

## 1.2   The Joy of Dance for Older Adults

The joy of dance for older adults is a celebration of movement that transcends the physical and resonates deeply with the emotional and social dimensions of well-being. Dance, with its rhythmic cadence and expressive forms, offers a unique avenue for seniors to experience a renewed sense of vitality and self-expression.

At its core, dance is an art form that allows individuals to connect with their bodies in a way that is both liberating and invigorating. For older adults, who may contend with the effects of aging on mobility and flexibility, dance provides a means to rediscover the potential and grace of their bodies. It's an opportunity to move freely, fostering a sense of autonomy and accomplishment.

Beyond the physical, the joy of dance lies in its ability to uplift the spirit. Engaging in dance releases endorphins, the body's natural mood enhancers, promoting a sense of happiness and reducing stress. The rhythmic patterns and expressive movements become a form of creative expression, allowing seniors to communicate and connect with their emotions in a positive and constructive way.

Dance is also a social endeavor, creating avenues for meaningful connections. Whether participating in group dance classes or engaging in partner dances, older adults can build a sense of community and camaraderie. The shared experience of moving to music fosters connections, breaks down social barriers, and cultivates a supportive environment.

In the twilight years, the joy of dance becomes a source of timeless delight. It's a testament to the enduring spirit within each individual, reminding them that the capacity for joy and self-expression knows no age. Through dance, older adults not only revel in the pleasure of movement but also discover a profound and lasting source of joy that contributes to a rich and fulfilling life.

# 1.3 Purpose and Scope of the Guide

The purpose of this guide is to empower seniors aged 60 and above to embrace the world of dance as a holistic means of enhancing their physical health, cognitive well-being, and overall quality of life. By navigating through the comprehensive information provided, readers will gain insights into the benefits of dance, safety precautions, and practical tips for incorporating dance routines into their daily lives.

The scope of the guide encompasses a diverse range of aspects related to dance for seniors. It starts with elucidating the multifaceted advantages of dance, touching upon physical fitness, cognitive stimulation, and emotional well-being. Safety precautions are thoroughly explored to ensure that seniors can enjoy the benefits of dance without compromising their health.

The guide delves into the practical aspects of dance, including warm-up exercises, simple dance moves, and the choreography of basic routines tailored to the unique needs and abilities of older adults. It provides guidance on music selection, emphasizing its motivational and expressive role in the dance experience.

Additionally, the guide recognizes the social dimension of dance for seniors. It explores the potential for building communities, whether through group classes, partner dances, or other social aspects of dance participation.

To enrich the reader's journey, the guide also offers resources for further exploration, success stories to inspire, and frequently asked questions to address common concerns. Ultimately, the purpose and scope of this guide converge to illuminate the transformative power of dance in the lives of seniors, fostering a sense of joy, community, and continued personal growth.

# 1.4 Purpose of Dance for Seniors

Dancing serves elders' needs in ways that go well beyond simple exercise. It is a multifaceted, holistic approach to well-being that improves people's lives.

1.  Physical Well-Being: Dancing is a fun way to work out that improves flexibility, cardiovascular health, and general mobility. It supports the preservation of bone density and joint health, two essential elements for elders navigating the aging process.

2.  Mental Well-being: Engaging in dance has profound cognitive benefits. It stimulates the brain, improving memory, concentration, and cognitive function. The rhythmic and patterned nature of dance can be a powerful tool in mitigating the risk of cognitive decline and promoting mental acuity.

3.  Emotional Expression: Dance provides a channel for emotional expression and creativity. Seniors can express themselves through movement, fostering a sense of accomplishment and joy. This emotional outlet contributes significantly to mental and emotional well-being.

4.  Social Interaction: Participating in dance classes or group dance activities facilitates social connections. Seniors can form new friendships, share experiences, and build a supportive community. The social aspect of dance is a powerful antidote to feelings of isolation or loneliness.

5. Improved Mood and Stress Reduction: The endorphins released during physical activity contribute to an improved mood. Dance can be a source of stress relief, helping seniors to unwind, relax, and enjoy the present moment.

6. Balance and Coordination: Many dance styles involve movements that enhance balance and coordination. This is particularly beneficial for seniors as it helps prevent falls and maintains their overall sense of stability.

7. Sense of Purpose: Engaging in regular dance routines provides seniors with a sense of purpose and accomplishment. It offers a structured and enjoyable activity that contributes positively to their daily lives.

Dancing for seniors aims to improve their quality of life primarily through four channels: physical health promotion, brain stimulation, emotional well-being, and social environment support. It goes beyond the physical motions to become a wellspring of happiness, fulfilment, and kinship during the golden years of life.

# Chapter 2

# Benefits of Dance for Seniors

## 2.1 Physical Health Benefits

Seniors who dance can get a variety of physical health advantages:

1. Cardiovascular Fitness: Dancing is a great cardiovascular exercise, whether you're dancing a slow waltz or a vivacious two-step. It enhances blood circulation and raises heart rate, supporting a robust cardiovascular system.

2. Range of Motion and Flexibility: Dancing incorporates a range of motions that engage and stretch various muscle groups, improving range of motion and promoting flexibility. For seniors in particular, this is crucial to avoid joint problems and stiffness.

3. Strength and Endurance of Muscles: The diverse motions used in dance routines contribute to the development and toning of

muscles across the body. Enhancing strength and endurance is beneficial for daily tasks and preserving one's independence.

4. Bone Density Preservation: Dance moves that require weight bearing, such jumping or some footwork-based dance forms, help to preserve bone density. Osteoporosis and other problems relating to the bones must be avoided by doing this.

5. Better Posture: Good posture and body alignment are frequently emphasized in dance. Frequent engagement can improve general spine health, lower the chance of back issues, and improve posture.

6. Calorie Burning and Weight Management: Seniors who participate in dance classes can burn a substantial amount of calories, contingent on the level of intensity of the dance type. This promotes a healthy lifestyle in general and aids with weight management.

7. Improved Balance and synchronization: Dancing tests balance and calls for

synchronization between various body parts. Seniors can particularly benefit from this as it increases general stability and reduces the risk of falls.

8. Pain Relieving: Dancing's flowing, rhythmic motions have the potential to naturally reduce pain. It can release tension from joints and muscles, relieving common aging-related aches and pains.

9. Increased Energy Levels: Regular dance sessions can boost energy levels. The combination of physical activity, music, and social interaction creates an environment that invigorates the body and mind.

10. Improved Circulation: The continuous and varied movements in dance stimulate blood flow, promoting better circulation. This is essential for delivering oxygen and nutrients to various parts of the body.

Incorporating dance into a senior's routine can contribute significantly to their physical health, offering a holistic approach to maintaining vitality and well-being.

## 2.2 Mental Health Benefits

Engaging in dance offers a range of mental health benefits for seniors:

1.  Cognitive Stimulation:

Learning and remembering dance routines stimulate the brain, enhancing cognitive functions such as memory and problem-solving. This mental engagement can contribute to maintaining cognitive health.

2.  Mood Elevation:

The physical activity associated with dance releases endorphins, often referred to as "feel-good" hormones. This natural mood elevation can help alleviate symptoms of depression and anxiety, promoting a positive emotional state.

3.  Stress Reduction:

Dance provides a creative and enjoyable outlet for releasing stress. The combination of music, movement, and social interaction can help seniors unwind, reducing overall stress levels.

4.  Increased Confidence and Self-esteem:
Mastering dance moves and participating in group activities can boost confidence and self-esteem. Seniors often gain a sense of accomplishment, positively impacting their perception of self-worth.

5.  Emotional Expression:
Dance allows seniors to express themselves physically and emotionally. Whether it's the joy of movement or a more contemplative expression, dancing provides an outlet for emotions, contributing to emotional well-being.

6.  Social Connection:
Participating in dance classes or group dances fosters social interaction. Building connections with others in a supportive environment helps combat feelings of loneliness and isolation, promoting mental health.

7.  Mind-Body Connection:
The mind-body connection inherent in dance is powerful. Being present in the moment, concentrating on movements, and syncing with music contribute to mindfulness, promoting mental clarity and focus.

8.  Neuroplasticity:
Dance, with its varying choreography, challenges the brain and promotes neuroplasticity — the brain's ability to reorganize itself. This can be particularly beneficial for seniors in maintaining cognitive flexibility.

9.  Improved Sleep Patterns:
Regular physical activity, such as dance, can positively influence sleep patterns. Improved sleep quality is associated with better mental health and cognitive function.

10. Sense of Purpose:
Engaging in dance provides seniors with a sense of purpose. Having regular activities to look forward to and goals to achieve, even if they're dance-related, contributes to a positive outlook on life.

By addressing both physical and mental aspects, dance emerges as a holistic practice that nurtures the overall well-being of seniors, promoting cognitive vitality, emotional resilience, and a positive outlook on life.

## 2.3 Social Benefits

Participating in dance provides seniors with a range of social benefits:

1.  Community Building:

Dance classes and group sessions create a sense of community among seniors. Shared experiences and a common interest in dance contribute to the formation of supportive social networks.

2.  Friendship and Connection:

Engaging in dance fosters the opportunity to build new friendships. Shared moments on the dance floor often translate into deeper connections, offering companionship and a sense of belonging.

3.  Reduced Isolation:

For seniors who may be at risk of isolation, dance becomes a social lifeline. Regular interactions in dance settings help combat loneliness and provide meaningful social engagement.

4.  Teamwork and Collaboration:

Partner dances or group routines encourage teamwork and collaboration. Seniors work together to master choreography, strengthening social bonds and promoting a sense of unity.

5.  Communication Skills:

Dance often involves non-verbal communication through movement. Seniors can enhance their communication skills by expressing themselves on the dance floor, fostering a unique form of interaction.

6.  Support System:

The social connections formed through dance can serve as a valuable support system. Seniors share not only the joy of dancing but also provide emotional support to one another, creating a nurturing environment.

7. Celebration of Diversity:

Dance classes attract individuals from various backgrounds and experiences. Seniors have the opportunity to celebrate diversity, fostering an inclusive and enriching social environment.

8. Social Events and Celebrations:

Dance communities often organize social events and celebrations. This provides seniors with occasions to come together, celebrate milestones, and enjoy each other's company beyond the dance floor.

9. Sense of Belonging:

Dancing creates a sense of belonging to a larger group. Seniors feel connected to others who share a passion for movement, contributing to a feeling of inclusivity and community.

10. Emotional Support:

During challenging times, the social connections established through dance offer emotional support. Whether celebrating achievements or providing comfort during difficulties, these connections become a valuable part of seniors' lives.

In essence, the social benefits of dance for seniors extend far beyond the physical movements. Dance becomes a conduit for building relationships, fostering a sense of community, and enhancing the overall social well-being of seniors.

# Chapter 3

# Considerations for Seniors' Health

## 3.1 Physical Limitations

When introducing dance to seniors, it's important to acknowledge and work with their physical limitations. Typical physical restrictions consist of:

1. Joint Problems: Older adults may have pain or stiffness in their knees and hips, among other joints. Dance routines should be modified with an emphasis on low-impact moves and moderate stretches to reduce the strain on these joints.

2. Balance Concerns: Issues with balance are common among seniors. Dance routines should incorporate movements that enhance balance, and seniors may benefit from holding onto a sturdy support or partner for stability.

3. Limited Range of Motion: Reduced flexibility and range of motion can be a challenge. Dance routines should include gradual stretches to improve flexibility, and modifications may be necessary to accommodate limited range of motion.

4. Cardiovascular Conditions: Seniors with cardiovascular conditions may need to approach dance with caution. It's essential to consult with a healthcare professional to ensure that dance routines align with their cardiovascular health and stamina.

5. Osteoporosis: Those with osteoporosis require careful consideration, as certain dance movements may pose a risk to bone health. Low-impact dances and activities that avoid excessive twisting or impact are advisable.

6. Muscle Weakness: Muscle weakness, especially in the lower body, is common. Dance routines should gradually build strength, with a focus on exercises that target specific muscle groups while avoiding excessive strain.

7. Respiratory Issues: Seniors with respiratory issues may need modifications in dance routines to accommodate their breathing capacity. Slow-paced dances or routines with designated rest intervals may be more suitable.

8. Sensitivity to Loud Music: Some seniors may have sensitivity to loud music. Dance classes or sessions should consider using lower volume levels or providing ear protection to make the experience more comfortable.

9. Chronic Pain Conditions: Chronic pain conditions, such as arthritis, may affect a senior's ability to engage in certain dance movements. Dance routines should be tailored to minimize impact on painful areas while promoting gentle movement.

10. Mobility Aids: Seniors who use mobility aids, such as canes or walkers, may need adaptations in dance routines. Seated dances or those that allow for the use of mobility aids should be incorporated.

Understanding and addressing these physical limitations with empathy and careful planning ensures that dance routines are not only enjoyable but also safe and beneficial for seniors. Before starting any dance program, consultation with healthcare professionals is advisable to create a personalized approach that considers individual needs and conditions.

## 3.2 Medical Consultation

Medical consultations are paramount before seniors embark on a dance program, ensuring their safety and well-being. Key considerations for medical consultations include:

1. Overall Health Assessment:

A comprehensive health assessment by a healthcare professional is crucial. This assessment should cover cardiovascular health, joint function, respiratory capacity, and any existing medical conditions.

2. Cardiovascular Health:

Seniors should discuss their cardiovascular health with a healthcare provider, especially if they have a history of heart conditions or high blood pressure.

This ensures that dance routines align with their cardiovascular capacity.

### 3. Joint and Muscular Health:

Assessing joint and muscular health is essential, particularly if seniors experience arthritis, joint pain, or muscle weakness. Medical professionals can provide guidance on suitable dance movements and adaptations.

### 4. Respiratory Capacity:

Seniors with respiratory conditions should consult with healthcare providers to determine the appropriateness of dance activities. Modifications may be necessary to accommodate their breathing capacity.

### 5. Balance and Coordination:

Evaluating balance and coordination is crucial, especially for seniors at risk of falls. Healthcare professionals can recommend specific exercises and dance modifications to enhance balance and coordination.

6. Bone Health:
Seniors with osteoporosis or other bone-related concerns need careful consideration. Medical consultations can guide the development of dance routines that support bone health without posing a risk of fractures.

7. Existing Medical Conditions:
Discussion about any existing medical conditions, such as diabetes or chronic pain, is essential. Healthcare professionals can provide insights into how dance may impact these conditions and suggest adjustments accordingly.

8. Medication Review:
Seniors should provide a list of medications they are taking. Certain medications may influence physical activity, and healthcare professionals can offer advice on how dance may interact with these medications.

9. Mobility Aids:
If seniors use mobility aids, such as canes or walkers, healthcare providers can offer guidance on how to integrate these aids into dance routines safely.

10. Customized Recommendations:
Based on the assessment, healthcare professionals can provide personalized recommendations, including the frequency and intensity of dance sessions, specific movements to focus on or avoid, and any precautions to be taken.

Medical consultations create a foundation for seniors to engage in dance activities safely, ensuring that the chosen routines align with their individual health profiles. Regular check-ins with healthcare professionals can also help monitor progress and make necessary adjustments as needed.

# Chapter 4

# Choosing Appropriate Music

## 4.1 Tempo and Rhythm

When it comes to senior dancing, the music's tempo and rhythm are crucial in fostering a positive and pleasurable experience. Here are some ways that rhythm and tempo enhance a satisfying dance experience:

1. Engagement and Motivation:
A moderate tempo with a clear rhythm can be motivating for seniors. It provides a steady pace that encourages movement without feeling rushed, fostering an engaging and enjoyable dance experience.

2. Adaptability to Movement Abilities:
The tempo should be adaptable to the participants' movement abilities. A slower tempo may be suitable for seniors who are just starting or have mobility challenges, allowing them to follow the rhythm comfortably.

3.  Physical Benefits:
The tempo influences the intensity of physical activity. Upbeat tempos can contribute to cardiovascular exercise, while slower tempos are suitable for gentle movements, promoting flexibility and joint mobility.

4.  Mood and Emotional Response:
The rhythm and tempo of music can evoke specific emotions. Upbeat and lively rhythms often contribute to a positive and joyful atmosphere, while slower tempos may create a more relaxed and contemplative mood.

5.  Variety and Interest:
Incorporating a variety of tempos and rhythms within a dance routine adds interest and engagement. This diversity keeps participants stimulated and encourages them to explore different movements.

6.  Safety and Comfort:
The tempo should align with participants' comfort levels and safety. Too fast a tempo may lead to

discomfort or a feeling of being overwhelmed, while too slow may not provide enough stimulation.

7. Music Selection:
Tailoring the music to the preferences of the participants is essential. Familiar tunes with a clear rhythm can enhance the overall experience, making it more enjoyable and relatable.

8. Social Interaction:
The tempo influences the style of dance and social interaction. Upbeat tempos may encourage more energetic and social dances, while slower tempos can create a conducive environment for partnered or group dances.

9. Accessibility for All:
Choosing music with a tempo that accommodates a range of abilities ensures inclusivity. Dance routines can be adapted to suit participants with varying levels of mobility, allowing everyone to participate comfortably.

10. Cultural Considerations:
Considering the cultural background and preferences of the participants is important. Different cultures

may have specific rhythms and tempos associated with traditional dances, adding cultural richness to the experience.

In conclusion, the senior dancing activity's overall success and satisfaction are influenced by the tempo and rhythm of the music. Seniors can have a dance experience that is not only physically healthy but also emotionally and socially stimulating when these factors are carefully taken into account.

## 4.2 Familiarity and Enjoyment

For elders to have a positive and interesting dancing experience, familiarity and enjoyment are essential:

1. Emotional Connection: Seniors can feel a connection when you play music they are familiar with. Songs that are associated with their time period or cultural background arouse sentimental feelings and bring back memories.

2. Motivation for Participation: Seniors who enjoy dancing are sometimes inspired to do

so by well-known songs. Dancing becomes more fun when people actively participate with the music they recognise and connect with.

3. Increased Comfort and Confidence: Seniors' comfort levels are raised and their confidence to move freely is boosted when they dance to music they are familiar with. Getting the beat and lyrics right makes you feel at ease, which adds to the happy and carefree vibe.

4. Cultural Relevance: Considering the participants' cultural backgrounds guarantees that the music chosen is both well-known and appropriate for the group. This gives the dancing experience an additional dimension of authenticity and inclusion.

5. Variety to Fit Preferences: Different tastes are catered to by providing a range of well-known music genres. Having options makes it easier for seniors to select dances that suit their preferences, whether it be Latin, swing, or ballroom.

6. Inspires Singing Along: Singing along to well-known songs is frequently an impromptu activity. This gives the dancing session a new level of excitement by stimulating the body and the voice through several senses.

7. Cognitive Stimulation and Memory Recall: Dancing to well-known music can improve memory recall. Seniors may benefit from the cognitive stimulation that comes from moving and listening to music together because it engages the brain.

8. Social Connection: When people are familiar with the same tunes, it helps them feel more connected to each other. The social side of the event is improved, whether you're dancing to your favorite song or thinking back on past experiences.

9. Customization of Dance Routine: Teachers or coordinators can make dance routines unique by basing them on the music preferences of the participants. This personalization puts a

nice finishing touch and shows that the people involved are taken into mind.

10. Long-Term involvement: Dancing to well-known music is enjoyable and helps foster long-term involvement. Seniors who find dancing regularly fun and meaningful are more likely to maintain their enthusiasm in the activity.

In conclusion, adding well-known and entertaining music to senior dancing classes fosters a supportive, emotionally rich, and inclusive setting that is inclusive of all cultures. It draws on the power of well-known songs and treasured memories to improve not just the physical benefits of dance but also the general well-being of elders.

## 4.3 Music Accessibility

Ensuring music accessibility is crucial for creating an inclusive and enjoyable dance experience for seniors. Considerations for making music accessible include:

1.  Varied Music Genres:

Provide a diverse selection of music genres to accommodate different tastes and preferences. This ensures that seniors can enjoy dances ranging from classic ballroom to contemporary tunes, promoting inclusivity.

2.  Cultural Diversity:

Recognize and include music from various cultural backgrounds. This adds richness to the dance experience and ensures that participants from diverse cultures feel represented and engaged.

3.  Clear Audio Quality:

Ensure that the audio quality is clear and easily understandable. Seniors may have varying levels of hearing ability, and quality sound enhances the overall enjoyment and comprehension of the music.

4.  Volume Control:

Have the ability to adjust the volume according to the participants' comfort. Some seniors may prefer a lower volume, while others may enjoy a slightly higher volume for a more immersive experience.

5.  Live Music Options:
If feasible, consider incorporating live music. Live performances can create a dynamic and interactive atmosphere, providing a unique and engaging experience for seniors.

6.  Accessible Devices:
Make sure that the devices used to play music are user-friendly and accessible. Large, clearly labeled buttons and simple controls can facilitate independent use for seniors.

7.  Lyric Display:
If the dance involves singing along, display lyrics on a screen or provide printed copies. This helps seniors follow along and actively participate in the musical aspect of the dance.

8.  Music Streaming Services:
Utilize music streaming services that offer a wide range of songs. This allows for flexibility in selecting and adapting playlists based on the preferences of the participants.

9.  Educational Components:
Incorporate educational elements about the music being played. Sharing information about the artist, era, or cultural context enhances the participants' connection to the music.


10. Feedback and Preferences:
Regularly seek feedback from participants regarding music preferences. This ensures that the chosen music aligns with their tastes, making the dance sessions more enjoyable and tailored to their preferences.


11. Adaptability to Different Devices:
Ensure that the music source is compatible with various devices, such as smartphones, tablets, or specialized audio equipment. This accommodates different technological preferences and capabilities.


12. Preparation for Virtual Sessions:
If conducting virtual dance sessions, provide clear instructions on accessing the music online. Familiarize participants with any virtual platforms used and ensure they have the necessary tools to participate remotely.

By addressing these aspects of music accessibility, dance organizers can create an inclusive and engaging environment, allowing seniors to fully enjoy the physical, mental, and social benefits of dance.

# Chapter 5

# Simple Dance Moves for Seniors

## 5. 1 Low-Impact Steps

For elders to dance in safety and enjoyment, low-impact steps must be incorporated into routines. The following low-impact exercises are appropriate for seniors:

1. Side Steps:

Encourage seniors to step side to side, maintaining a gentle and controlled pace. This movement promotes lateral mobility without placing excessive strain on joints.

2. Marching in Place:

Simple marching in place allows for rhythmic movement without the need for extensive travel. It provides cardiovascular benefits while being low impact on joints.

3.  Toe Taps:

Lift one foot at a time to tap the toes on the floor. This low-impact movement helps with balance and engages leg muscles without the need for intense jumping or lifting.

4.  Heel Touches:

Encourage seniors to touch their heels to the floor alternately while maintaining a steady rhythm. This movement engages calf muscles and promotes flexibility.

5.  Grapevine Step:

The grapevine step involves crossing one foot over the other and then stepping to the side. It's a smooth and controlled movement that promotes coordination and lateral mobility.

6.  Box Step:

With a focus on precision and control, the box step involves stepping forward, to the side, back, and then to the other side. It's a structured and low-impact movement suitable for seniors.

7.  Knee Lifts:
Lift one knee at a time in a controlled manner. This low-impact step engages the core and leg muscles, promoting balance and flexibility.

8.  Swaying Hips:
Incorporate gentle hip sways from side to side. This movement adds a playful element to dance routines and promotes flexibility in the hip area.

9.  Arm Circles:
Engage the upper body with low-impact arm circles. Seniors can rotate their arms in both directions, promoting shoulder mobility and flexibility.

10. Slow Turns:
Introduce slow turns without sudden twists. This adds variety to the dance routine while allowing seniors to practice balance and coordination.

11. Slow Waltz Steps:
Teach basic slow waltz steps, emphasizing the gliding nature of the dance. This classic ballroom step is graceful and gentle on joints.

12. Seated Marching:

For seniors with limited mobility, seated marching provides an excellent low-impact option. It promotes circulation and engages the leg muscles while sitting comfortably.

13. Chair Dancing:
Utilize a chair for support, incorporating seated dance movements such as swaying, tapping, and arm motions. This makes dance accessible for seniors with mobility challenges.

14. Side Leg Lifts:
Lift one leg to the side in a controlled manner, engaging the hip and outer thigh muscles. This low-impact movement promotes leg strength and flexibility.

15. Slow Cha-Cha Steps:
Introduce slow cha-cha steps with a focus on controlled footwork. This rhythmic movement is suitable for seniors and adds a lively element to dance routines.

These low-impact dancing moves make for a safe and fun experience when creating senior dance routines, encouraging physical activity while putting joint health and comfort first.

## 5. 2 Arm Movements

Incorporating expressive and controlled arm movements adds flair and engagement to dance routines for seniors. Here are some arm movements suitable for a senior-friendly dance session:

1. Arm Swings: Gentle arm swings from side to side promote flexibility in the shoulders. Seniors can perform these movements at their own pace, enjoying the rhythmic flow.

2. Side Reaches: Encourage seniors to reach one arm to the side, creating elongation through the torso. Alternate between arms for a graceful and stretching movement.

3. Upward Reaches: Lift both arms overhead in a slow and controlled manner. This movement stretches the upper body and engages the core muscles.

4.  Circle Arms: Perform slow, circular arm movements in both clockwise and counterclockwise directions. This gentle rotation promotes mobility in the shoulder joints.

5.  Bicep Curls: Incorporate bicep curls by bending and straightening the elbows. Seniors can hold onto light weights or water bottles for added resistance if they feel comfortable doing so.

6.  Floating Arms: Create a sense of floating by moving the arms in a fluid, wave-like motion. This adds a graceful and flowing quality to the dance routine.

7.  Diagonal Reaches: Combine arm movements with diagonal reaches, extending one arm diagonally across the body. This engages the obliques and adds variety to the routine.

8.  Palm Presses: Press the palms together in front of the chest and then extend the arms outward. This movement promotes chest opening and stretching.

9. Figure-Eight Arms: Draw figure-eight patterns with the arms, emphasizing smooth and controlled movements. This adds a playful and rhythmic element to the dance.

10. Wrist Rolls: Rotate the wrists in circular motions, promoting flexibility and mobility in the wrists and forearms. This is particularly beneficial for seniors with arthritis.

11. Boxing Punches: Perform slow and controlled boxing punches, extending one arm at a time. This movement engages the arm muscles and adds an element of fun to the routine.

12. Pendulum Arms: Swing the arms gently from side to side, mimicking the motion of a pendulum. This rhythmic movement encourages coordination and balance.

13. Seated Arm Marches: For seniors who are seated, incorporate arm marches by lifting the

arms in a marching motion. This adds an aerobic element while seated.

14. Twisting Arms: Combine arm movements with torso twists for a coordinated upper-body workout. This engages the core and promotes flexibility in the spine.

15. Partner Arm Gestures: In group settings, incorporate partner arm gestures, such as linking arms or synchronized movements. This fosters social interaction and a sense of connection among participants.

When integrating arm movements into dance routines for seniors, it's important to prioritize comfort and safety. Encourage participants to move within their range of motion, and provide variations to accommodate different abilities. These arm movements contribute to a well-rounded and enjoyable dance experience, promoting both physical activity and artistic expression.

# Chapter 6

# Partner or Group Dances

## 6.1 Simple Partner Dance Ideas

Seniors can benefit from easy partner dance concepts that improve social interaction and give dancing a fun new dimension. Here are a few simple and flexible partner dance suggestions:

1. Hand-in-Hand Waltz: This is a basic waltz movement in which partners hold hands and sway gently back and forth. Stress the flowing elegance and invite couples to share the song.

2. Side-Step Swing: Partners face one another and move in unison as they step side to side. This relaxed swing dance step keeps the movement comfortable and regular, yet it still permits social engagement.

3.  Mirror Dance:  Partners face one another and alternately lead movements in the mirror dance. A basic step is started by one partner, and the other partner imitates the motion. This promotes synchronization and a feeling of unity.

4.  Gently Salsa: Show couples how to do a fundamental salsa step, focusing on tiny side steps and hip motions. The emphasis is on having fun and fostering a social environment.

5.  Circle Dancing: Two people hold hands and circle each other. This group dance fosters camaraderie among participants and promotes communication with several partners.

6.  Slow Two-Step: Partners can engage in a slow two-step, moving forward and backward together. This uncomplicated dance allows for conversation while enjoying the rhythmic steps.

7. Shoulder Tap Jive: Partners stand side by side, and one partner lightly taps the other's shoulder to signal a quick change of direction. This adds an element of playfulness to the dance.

8. Rocking Chair Swing: Partners face each other and gently rock back and forth in a synchronized motion. This simple and intimate movement creates a soothing dance experience.

9. Hand Clap Cha-Cha: Partners incorporate hand claps into a basic cha-cha step. This rhythmic dance adds a sense of play and engagement between partners.

10. Back-and-Forth Polka: Partners face each other and move forward and backward in a simple polka step. This lively dance adds a touch of energy to the routine.

11. Partner Promenade: Partners link arms and promenade around the dance space. This classic ballroom-style movement encourages a sense of elegance and coordination.

12. Circles and Turns Foxtrot: Partners move in circles and incorporate gentle turns in a foxtrot-like fashion. This introduces variety while maintaining simplicity.

13. Simple Box Step: Partners can learn a basic box step, moving forward, side, together, back, side, together. This foundational step is easy to follow and allows for creative variations.

14. Holding Hands Jig: Partners hold hands and perform a light and easy jig, incorporating small hops and rhythmic footwork. This joyful dance adds a playful element to the routine.

Make ease of use, comfort, and the enjoyment of group dancing your top priorities when instructing seniors in partner dances. Promote flexibility and adjustments in accordance with participants' skill levels to create a welcoming and upbeat dance atmosphere.

# 6.2 Group Choreography Options

Creating group choreography for seniors involves selecting movements that are inclusive, enjoyable, and considerate of varying abilities. Here are some group choreography options suitable for seniors:

1.  Circle Dance:

Form a large circle, and participants move in a coordinated manner, following simple steps. This fosters a sense of unity and allows for social interaction as they dance together.

2.  Line Dance:

Introduce easy-to-follow line dance steps that the group can perform in unison. This genre often features repetitive movements and provides a structured yet enjoyable experience.

3.  Swinging Waltz:

Create a group waltz where participants link arms and sway together in a gentle waltz rhythm. This classic ballroom dance encourages collaboration and shared movement.

4.  Folk Dance Medley:
Incorporate a medley of simple folk dance steps from various cultures. This adds cultural diversity to the choreography and allows participants to explore different dance styles.

5.  Chair Dance Routine:
Design a dance routine that incorporates the use of chairs. Seated or standing, participants can engage in movements that utilize the stability of chairs, ensuring accessibility for all.

6.  Partnered Square Dance:
Adapt square dance formations to include partnered movements. This adds a social element to the traditional square dance and encourages teamwork.

7.  Celebratory Conga Line:
Incorporate a lively conga line into the choreography, where participants follow a leader in a celebratory procession. This adds a festive and interactive element to the dance routine.

8.  Rhythmic Tap Routine:
Create a tap dance routine with simple rhythmic footwork. Use percussion instruments or tap shoes

to enhance the auditory experience while maintaining a low-impact approach.

9. Social Salsa Circle:
Form a circle and introduce basic salsa steps that participants can perform together. This lively and rhythmic dance style encourages interaction and creates a vibrant atmosphere.

10. Gentle Jazzercise:
Develop a choreography that incorporates elements of jazzercise, focusing on easy-to-follow movements that promote cardiovascular health and overall well-being.

11. Nature-Inspired Movements:
Design a dance routine inspired by nature, incorporating flowing and graceful movements that mimic elements like leaves rustling or waves gently rolling. This provides a calming and artistic experience.

12. Memory Lane Dance:
Choreograph movements that reflect iconic dances from different decades. This nostalgic journey

through dance styles allows participants to reminisce and enjoy a variety of movements.

13. Mirror Dance Improvisation:
Create a segment where participants pair up and take turns leading and following movements. This improvisational approach encourages creativity and adaptability within the group.

# Chapter 7

# Seated Dance Options

## 7. 1 Benefits of Seated Dancing

Seated dance offers a range of physical, mental, and social benefits, making it a highly accessible and enjoyable activity, especially for seniors. Here are some key benefits of seated dance:

1. Improved Mobility: Seated dance routines incorporate gentle movements that promote joint flexibility and muscle mobility. This is particularly beneficial for seniors with limited mobility or those who may find standing for extended periods challenging.

2. Enhanced Cardiovascular Health: Engaging in rhythmic seated movements can elevate the heart rate, providing cardiovascular benefits without putting excessive strain on the joints. This contributes to improved circulation and heart health.

3. Muscle Engagement: Seated dance involves a variety of arm, leg, and core movements, providing a full-body workout. It helps seniors maintain muscle strength and endurance, supporting overall physical function.

4. Joint Protection: The seated position reduces the impact on joints, making it a safe option for individuals with arthritis or joint pain. Seated dance allows participants to enjoy movement without exacerbating existing joint conditions.

5. Balance and Stability: Seated dance routines can include exercises that enhance balance and stability. These movements contribute to fall prevention and help seniors maintain a sense of equilibrium.

6. Pain Management: Seated dance can act as a gentle form of pain management. The rhythmic and controlled movements may alleviate tension in muscles and joints, providing relief from common aches and pains associated with aging.

7. Improved Posture: Seated dance often emphasizes maintaining good posture. Engaging in movements while seated encourages participants to sit upright, contributing to better spinal alignment and reduced strain on the back.

8. Enhanced Mood and Mental Well-being: The combination of music and movement stimulates the release of endorphins, promoting a positive mood. Seated dance provides a creative outlet for self-expression, contributing to mental well-being and stress reduction.

9. Cognitive Stimulation: Learning and following seated dance routines can stimulate cognitive functions. It requires concentration, memory, and coordination, providing a cognitively engaging activity that supports brain health.

10. Social Interaction: Seated dance can be done individually or in group settings, fostering social interaction. Group sessions offer a

sense of community, allowing participants to share the joy of movement in a supportive environment.

11. Accessible for All Fitness Levels: Seated dance is adaptable to various fitness levels and physical abilities. It accommodates individuals with different mobility challenges, making it an inclusive activity for a diverse group of seniors.

12. Increased Energy Levels: Participating in seated dance can boost energy levels. The combination of music, movement, and social interaction creates an invigorating experience, leaving participants feeling more energized.

13. Flexibility Promotion: Seated dance routines often include gentle stretches that promote flexibility. Regular participation can contribute to maintaining or improving overall flexibility, reducing the risk of stiffness.

14. Emotional Expression: Seated dance allows seniors to express themselves physically and emotionally. Whether through hand movements, facial expressions, or body language, participants can convey emotions and creativity.

15. Enjoyable and Accessible Exercise: Seated dance provides a form of exercise that is enjoyable, accessible, and less intimidating than some traditional fitness activities. This increases the likelihood of sustained participation, promoting long-term health benefits.

Overall, seated dance is a versatile and inclusive activity that offers a holistic approach to well-being for seniors, addressing physical, mental, and social aspects of health.

## 7.2 Seated Dance Moves

Since seated dance routines are meant to be easy, accessible, and pleasurable, people of different levels of mobility can benefit from them. Senior dancing routines can incorporate the following seated dance moves:

1. March while sitting down: Raise one knee at a time in a marching motion. This exercise warms up the lower body, works the core, and increases circulation.

2. Shoulder Rolls: Rotate the shoulders in a circular motion, first forward and then backward. This helps release tension and promotes flexibility in the shoulder joints.

3. Arm Waves:

Extend arms forward and create a flowing wave motion by lifting and lowering the arms. This move enhances flexibility and coordination in the upper body.

4.  Toe Taps: Tap the toes on the floor alternately in a rhythmic pattern. This low-impact move engages the leg muscles and promotes circulation.

5.  Side Reaches:
Reach one arm at a time to the side, creating elongation through the torso. Alternate between arms for a graceful and stretching movement.

6.  Seated Twist: Gently twist the upper body from side to side while keeping the feet planted. This move promotes flexibility in the spine and engages the core.

7.  Knee Lifts: Lift one knee at a time toward the chest in a controlled manner. This seated marching variation targets the core and leg muscles.

8.  Hand Claps: Clap hands together in front, overhead, or to the sides, adding a rhythmic element to the seated dance routine.

9. Figure-Eight Arms: Draw figure-eight patterns with the arms, emphasizing smooth and controlled movements. This adds a playful and rhythmic element to the dance.

10. Seated Hip Swirls: Engage the hips by creating circular motions while remaining seated. This movement promotes flexibility and mobility in the hip joints.

11. Wrist Circles: Rotate the wrists in circular motions, promoting flexibility and mobility in the wrists and forearms.

12. Elbow Taps: Gently tap one elbow at a time to the opposite knee while sitting upright. This move engages the obliques and promotes a seated abdominal workout.

13. Seated Side Leg Lifts: Lift one leg at a time to the side in a controlled manner. This low-impact movement engages the hip and outer thigh muscles.

14. Open and Close: Extend both arms out to the sides and then bring them back together in front of the body. This move promotes chest opening and stretching.

15. Seated Rocking: Rock gently from side to side in the chair, following the rhythm of the music. This movement adds a soothing and rhythmic quality to the dance routine

These seated dance moves can be combined and adapted to create diverse and enjoyable routines for seniors. It's important to encourage participants to move within their comfort levels and modify movements based on individual abilities. The goal is to provide a fun and inclusive dance experience that promotes both physical and emotional well-being.

## 7.3 Adapting Traditional Dances for Seated Participants

Adapting traditional dances for seated participants involves modifying movements to accommodate individuals who may have mobility challenges. Here are adaptations for some popular traditional dances:

1. Seated Waltz:
- Participants can perform a simplified waltz by swaying gently side to side while seated.
- Incorporate hand movements, such as holding hands with a partner and moving arms in a flowing motion.

2. Seated Cha-Cha:
- Adapt the cha-cha by focusing on rhythmic hip movements while remaining seated.
- Participants can perform simple hand gestures and shoulder shimmies to add flair.

3. Seated Foxtrot:
- Simplify foxtrot steps by incorporating gentle side-to-side sways and arm movements.
- Partners can hold hands and move arms in coordination with the swaying motion.

4. Seated Swing:
- For a seated swing, participants can sway their upper bodies to the rhythm while tapping their feet or rocking their legs.

- Include hand-holding or hand-clapping movements for a social and interactive element.

5. Seated Salsa:
- Focus on upper body movements for a seated salsa, incorporating shoulder rolls, arm waves, and gentle torso twists.
- Encourage participants to use hand movements to mimic the lively spirit of salsa.

6. Seated Line Dance:
- Modify line dance steps to accommodate seated participants, emphasizing hand and arm movements.
- Encourage group synchronization with simple side-to-side sways and coordinated arm gestures.

7. Seated Tango:
- Simplify tango steps by focusing on dramatic arm movements and upper body expression.
- Encourage participants to engage in eye contact and convey emotion through seated gestures.

8.  Seated Polka:
- Adapt the polka by incorporating seated bouncing motions, emphasizing rhythmic upper body movements.
- Participants can hold hands or clap in coordination with the polka beat.

9.  Seated Jive:
- Modify jive steps by translating footwork into seated leg kicks and bouncing motions.
- Incorporate hand movements, such as jazz hands or finger snaps, for added energy.

10. Seated Irish Step Dance:
- Adapt Irish step dance by focusing on seated leg movements, such as tapping toes and heel lifts.
- Encourage participants to use hand and arm movements to express the dynamic nature of Irish dance.

11. Seated Square Dance:
- Simplify square dance steps by translating movements to seated sways and hand gestures.

- Encourage participants to interact with neighboring participants through coordinated hand movements.

12. Seated Bollywood Dance:
- Adapt Bollywood dance by incorporating seated hip shakes, hand gestures, and head movements.
- Use lively music and encourage participants to express the vibrant spirit of Bollywood.

When adapting traditional dances for seated participants, it's essential to prioritize comfort, safety, and enjoyment. Consider the mobility levels of participants and provide variations to accommodate diverse abilities.

Additionally, incorporating expressive hand and arm movements can enhance the seated dance experience, allowing participants to connect with the rhythm and spirit of each dance style.

# Chapter 8

# Incorporating Balance and Coordination

## 8.1 Balance Exercises

Improving balance is crucial for seniors to maintain mobility and reduce the risk of falls. Here are some balance exercises suitable for seniors:

1. Heel-to-Toe Walk:
   - Place one foot directly in front of the other in a straight line.
   - Walk in a heel-to-toe fashion, keeping the back foot's toes touching the front foot's heel with each step.

2. Single-Leg Stands:
   - Stand next to a sturdy surface for support.
   - Lift one leg and hold the position, aiming for 10-30 seconds.
   - Repeat on the other leg.

3. Chair Squats:
- Stand in front of a sturdy chair with feet hip-width apart.
- Lower the body into a seated position, then stand back up.
- Ensure the chair is there for support if needed.

4. Tightrope Walk:
- Imagine a straight line on the ground.
- Walk along this imaginary tightrope, lifting knees higher than usual for added challenge.

5. Side Leg Raises:
- Stand behind a sturdy chair with hands on the backrest.
- Lift one leg to the side, keeping it straight.
- Lower the leg back down and repeat on the other side.

6. Toe Raises:
- Stand with feet hip-width apart.
- Lift both heels off the ground, balancing on the toes, and then lower them back down.

7. Balance Exercises with Eyes Closed:

- Stand on one leg with eyes closed to challenge balance further.
- Use a sturdy surface for support if needed.

8. Tai Chi:
- Practice slow and controlled movements from tai chi, emphasizing weight shifts and balance.
- Many tai chi routines are designed to enhance balance and stability.

9. Back Leg Raises:
- Stand behind a sturdy chair, holding onto it for support.
- Lift one leg straight back, engaging the muscles in the buttocks and lower back.
- Lower the leg back down and repeat on the other side.

10. Marching in Place:
- Lift knees alternately, as if marching in place, engaging the core for stability.
- Use a wall or chair for support if needed.

11. Yoga Tree Pose:
- Stand on one leg and place the sole of the other foot against the inner thigh or calf.
- Bring hands together in front of the chest in a prayer position.
- Hold the pose for balance, then switch legs.

12. Weight Shifts:
- Stand with feet hip-width apart.
- Shift weight from one foot to the other, lifting the opposite foot slightly off the ground.

13. Clock Reaches:
- Imagine standing at the center of a clock.
- Reach one foot forward to 12 o'clock, then to 3 o'clock, 6 o'clock, and 9 o'clock.
- Repeat with the other foot.

14. Sit-to-Stand with Eyes Closed:
- Sit in a sturdy chair and stand up with eyes closed.
- Slowly sit back down, again with eyes closed, maintaining control.

15. Stork Stand:

- Stand on one leg and bring the opposite knee toward the chest.
- Hold the position for balance, then switch legs.

Seniors should consult with a healthcare professional before starting any new exercise routine, especially if they have pre-existing health conditions or concerns. These balance exercises can be adapted based on individual abilities and progressed gradually to improve stability over time.

## 8.2 Coordination Challenges

Improving coordination is important for overall mobility and preventing accidents, especially for seniors. Here are some exercises that can help address coordination challenges:

1. Ball Toss:
- Stand facing a partner or a wall.
- Toss a soft ball back and forth, varying the height and speed.
- This exercise improves hand-eye coordination.

2.  Balloon Tap:
- Tap a balloon in the air, keeping it aloft without letting it touch the ground.
- This activity enhances hand-eye coordination and motor skills.

3.  Hula Hooping:
- Use a lightweight hula hoop and practice keeping it spinning around the waist.
- This improves coordination and balance.

4.  Juggling Scarves:
- Start with lightweight scarves or tissues.
- Toss them in the air, aiming to keep multiple scarves moving simultaneously.
- This exercise enhances hand-eye coordination and focus.

5.  Catching and Throwing Rings:
- Toss lightweight plastic rings back and forth with a partner.
- This activity improves hand-eye coordination and depth perception.

6.  Walking the Line:

- Create a straight line on the floor with tape.
- Practice walking along the line, lifting knees higher for an added challenge.
- This helps with balance and coordination.

7. Cone Dribbling:
- Set up cones in a zigzag pattern.
- Dribble a small ball around the cones using a controlled and coordinated motion.
- This enhances coordination and agility.

8. Simon Says:
- Play a game of Simon Says with a variety of movements, such as clapping hands, tapping feet, or touching different body parts.
- This game challenges both physical and cognitive coordination.

9. Obstacle Course:
- Create a simple obstacle course using household items.
- Navigate through the course, incorporating activities like stepping over objects, turning around, or weaving through cones.
- This improves overall coordination and spatial awareness.

10. Mirror Movements:
- Stand facing a partner.
- One person initiates a series of simple movements, and the other person mirrors those movements.
- This activity enhances coordination and promotes social interaction.

11. Tap Dancing:
- Learn basic tap dance steps.
- The rhythmic nature of tap dancing helps improve coordination and timing.

12. Reaction Ball Bounces:
- Bounce a reaction ball against a wall and try to catch it as it comes back at unpredictable angles.
- This exercise improves reaction time and hand-eye coordination.

13. Rhythmic Clapping:
- Clap hands in different patterns, varying the rhythm and speed.
- This activity enhances hand coordination and rhythm perception.

14. Boxing Punches:
- Stand in a boxing stance and throw controlled punches into the air.
- This helps with hand-eye coordination and engages the entire body.

15. Dance-Based Activities:
- Participate in dance-based workouts that involve coordinated movements.
- Dance routines challenge coordination while providing an enjoyable and dynamic exercise.

These coordination exercises can be tailored to individual abilities and gradually progressed. It's important to start slowly, focus on proper form, and consult with a healthcare professional before beginning any new exercise regimen, especially for seniors or individuals with pre-existing health conditions.

# Chapter 9

# Safety Tips

## 9.1  Proper Footwear

Choosing the right footwear is crucial for seniors to ensure comfort, stability, and overall foot health. Here are some considerations for selecting proper footwear:

1. Comfortable Fit:
- Shoes should provide a snug but not tight fit. Look for styles with ample toe room to avoid crowding and potential discomfort.
- Ensure the shoe doesn't rub against any part of the foot, which could lead to blisters or sores.

2. Arch Support:
- Opt for shoes with good arch support to maintain proper foot alignment and reduce the risk of conditions like plantar fasciitis.

- Some shoes come with removable insoles, allowing for customization with orthotic inserts if needed.

3. Cushioning:
- Choose shoes with sufficient cushioning, especially in the heel and ball of the foot. This helps absorb shock during walking and provides added comfort.

4. Low Heel Height:
- Seniors should generally avoid shoes with high heels, as they can destabilize balance. Choose shoes with a low or flat heel for better stability.

5. Non-Slip Soles:
- Look for shoes with non-slip soles, especially important for preventing slips and falls. This is crucial for both indoor and outdoor activities.

6. Wide Base:
- Shoes with a wide base offer more stability, reducing the risk of tripping or losing balance. This is particularly important for seniors with mobility concerns.

7.  Adjustable Straps:

- Shoes with adjustable straps or closures (like Velcro) are easier to put on and take off. This is beneficial for seniors who may have difficulty tying laces.

8.  Lightweight Material:

- Lightweight shoes reduce the overall strain on the feet and legs. Heavy footwear can contribute to fatigue, making lightweight options preferable.

9.  Breathability:

- Choose shoes made from breathable materials to prevent moisture build-up and reduce the risk of fungal infections.
- Consider open-toe or open-heel designs for increased ventilation.

10. Proper Sizing:

Have feet measured regularly, as shoe sizes can change with age. Choose shoes that accommodate the larger foot if there is a size difference.

11. Easy to Clean:
Opt for shoes that are easy to clean. This is especially important for seniors who may have difficulty bending to clean their footwear regularly.

12. Diabetic-Friendly Options:
For individuals with diabetes, it's essential to choose shoes that provide extra cushioning, a seamless interior, and minimal pressure points to prevent complications.

13. Podiatrist Approval:
If there are specific foot concerns or conditions, consult with a podiatrist for personalized recommendations on suitable footwear.

14. Activity-Specific Shoes:
Consider the intended activity. Different shoes are designed for walking, running, or specific sports. Choose footwear tailored to the planned activities.

15. Regular Check for Wear and Tear:
Regularly inspect shoes for signs of wear and tear, such as worn-out soles or uneven wear patterns. Replace shoes as needed to maintain optimal support.

Remember that everyone's feet are unique, so personal comfort plays a significant role in selecting proper footwear. Regular foot check-ups, especially for seniors, can help address any emerging issues promptly.

## 9.2 Emergency Preparedness

Emergency preparedness is crucial for seniors to ensure their safety and well-being during unexpected situations. Here are key considerations for creating an emergency preparedness plan for seniors:

1. Emergency Contacts:
Maintain a list of emergency contacts, including family members, friends, neighbors, and healthcare providers. Share this list with someone you trust.

2. Medical Information:
Keep a record of medical information, including allergies, medications, and any existing health

conditions. Ensure this information is easily accessible in case of emergencies.

### 3. Communication Plan:

Establish a communication plan with family members and friends. Agree on a method to check in during emergencies and share important updates.

### 4. Evacuation Plan:

Identify evacuation routes and locations. Know where local shelters are located and have a plan for transportation in case evacuation becomes necessary.

### 5. Emergency Kit:

Prepare an emergency kit with essential items, including medications, a first aid kit, non-perishable food, water, flashlight, batteries, important documents, and comfort items.

### 6. Medication Management:

Ensure an adequate supply of medications is available. Consider having a medication list, including dosage instructions, in the emergency kit.

7. Medical Alert System:

If applicable, consider using a medical alert system that allows seniors to call for help in case of emergencies, especially if they live alone.

8. Assistance for Mobility Challenges:

Plan for assistance if there are mobility challenges. Know how to access transportation or arrange for help during evacuations.

9. Emergency Services Information:

Familiarize yourself with local emergency services, such as the nearest hospital, fire station, and police station. Save these numbers in your phone and keep a hard copy in your emergency kit.

10. Weather Alerts:

Stay informed about weather conditions and subscribe to weather alerts. Be aware of potential natural disasters common to your region.

11. Home Safety Measures:

Conduct a home safety assessment. Secure heavy furniture, install grab bars, and eliminate potential hazards to reduce the risk of injuries during emergencies.

12. Community Resources:
Identify local community resources that can provide assistance during emergencies, such as senior centers, community centers, or volunteer organizations.

13. Power Outage Preparedness:
Have a plan for power outages. Consider having alternative lighting sources, such as flashlights or lanterns, and a supply of non-perishable food that doesn't require cooking.

14. Transportation Alternatives:
If seniors no longer drive, establish alternative transportation options for emergencies. Coordinate with neighbors, friends, or local community services.

15. Regular Review and Practice:
Regularly review and update your emergency preparedness plan. Practice evacuation routes and procedures with family members or caregivers.

It's important for seniors and their caregivers to work together to create a comprehensive emergency preparedness plan tailored to individual needs. Regular communication and practice drills can enhance readiness and ensure a swift response during challenging situations.

# Chapter 10

# Creating a Weekly Routine

## 10.1 Frequency of Sessions

Depending on the type of activity, the person's level of fitness and health, and their preferences, different activities have different session frequencies. The following general rules apply to various session types:

1. Activity :
- Aim for at least 150 minutes per week, spread out throughout the week, of moderate-intensity aerobic activity.
- Every major muscle group should receive strength training exercises on two or more days per week.

2. Exercises for Flexibility and Balance:
- Try to fit in some balance exercises three times a week at the very least.

- To increase flexibility, stretch your main muscle groups at least twice or three times a week.

3. Movement or Dancing Sessions:
- Depending on your fitness level and personal preferences, do movement or dancing sessions many times a week.
- Think about adding these sessions to your weekly or daily schedule.

4. Cognitive Exercises:
- To keep the brain active, do cognitive exercises on a regular basis.
- Try to fit in puzzles, games, or picking up new abilities multiple times a week.

5. Social Activities:
- Participate in social activities regularly to promote mental well-being.
- This could include socializing with friends, joining clubs, or attending group events based on personal preferences.

6. Balance and Coordination Exercises:

- Practice balance and coordination exercises at least two to three times a week to enhance stability and prevent falls.

7. Emergency Preparedness Drills:
- Conduct emergency preparedness drills and reviews periodically to ensure familiarity with the plan.
- Review and update the plan as needed, but aim for at least once or twice a year.

8. Health Checkups:
- Schedule regular health checkups with healthcare providers as recommended.
- This may include routine checkups, eye exams, dental visits, and screenings for various health conditions.

9. Medication Management:
- Regularly review and manage medications with healthcare providers.
- This may involve daily or weekly routines for medication administration and monitoring.

10. Balance and Coordination Activities:

- Incorporate balance and coordination activities into daily routines.
- Consider brief sessions, such as practicing balancing while waiting for a meal to cook.

11. Relaxation Methods:
- To reduce tension, try deep breathing exercises or meditation as needed. You can do this once a week or several times a day.

12. Evaluation of Footwear:
- Make sure your shoes are comfortable and stable by regularly evaluating and updating them for safety and correct fit.
- This can be carried out as needed, but it's important to check frequently, particularly if the health of your feet changes.

It's critical to customize the number of sessions according to each person's preferences, health status, and any advice from medical professionals. A well-rounded strategy with a range of activities can enhance general wellbeing. Before beginning a new fitness or wellness programme, always get advice from healthcare professionals, especially if you're a senior and have pre-existing health issues.

# Conclusion

Establishing a well-rounded routine for seniors is paramount for their overall health, well-being, and safety. The frequency of sessions, whether for physical exercise, cognitive stimulation, social engagement, or emergency preparedness, should be personalized to individual needs and preferences. Striking a balance between aerobic exercises, strength training, balance activities, and flexibility exercises contributes to a comprehensive fitness regimen. Engaging in cognitive exercises, social activities, and relaxation techniques further enhances mental and emotional health.

Regular health checkups, medication management, and an emphasis on proper footwear underscore the importance of proactive healthcare. Incorporating seated dance or movement sessions provides a joyful and accessible means of staying active. Emergency preparedness drills, conducted periodically, ensure readiness for unexpected situations.

Ultimately, the key is to foster a holistic approach that addresses physical, mental, and social aspects of well-being. This multifaceted strategy not only enhances the quality of life for seniors but also contributes to their independence and resilience. As seniors and their caregivers collaborate on these routines, the goal is to create habits that promote longevity, vitality, and a fulfilling lifestyle. By embracing diverse activities and maintaining regular assessments, seniors can embark on a journey of continued well-being, adapting routines as needed to meet the evolving needs of aging gracefully.

# Quiz

1. What is the recommended minimum duration for moderate-intensity aerobic exercise per week?

A) 60 minutes

B) 90 minutes

C) 120 minutes

D) 150 minutes

2. How often should strength training activities be performed for all major muscle groups?

A) Once a week

B) Twice a week

C) Three times a week

D) Five times a week

3. Emergency Preparedness:

How frequently should emergency preparedness drills be conducted?

A) Monthly

B) Quarterly

C) Semi-annually

D) Annually

4. Social Activities:

Why are social activities important for seniors?

A) They improve physical health
B) They enhance mental well-being
C) They reduce the risk of isolation
D) All of the above

5. How often should seniors practice balance and coordination exercises?

A) Once a week
B) Two to three times a week
C) Daily
D) Only as needed

6. Why is regular footwear assessment important for seniors?

A) It ensures proper fit and comfort
B) It enhances stability and reduces the risk of falls
C) It promotes foot health
D) All of the above

7. Which of the following is a relaxation technique suitable for seniors?

A) Deep breathing
B) Meditation
C) Both A and B
D) Neither A nor B

8. How can seated dance sessions benefit seniors?

A) They provide cardiovascular exercise

B) They are accessible for various fitness levels

C) They promote social interaction

D) All of the above

9. What should seniors regularly review and manage with healthcare providers?

A) Exercise routines

B) Medications

C) Social activities

D) Dietary habits

10. Why is staying informed about weather conditions important for seniors?

A) To plan outdoor activities

B) To prepare for potential emergencies

C) To decide on clothing choices

D) Both A and B

11. Tai Chi Benefits:

How does practicing tai chi contribute to senior well-being?

A) It improves balance

B) It enhances flexibility

C) It promotes relaxation
D) All of the above

12. Why is it important to gradually progress fitness routines for seniors?
A) To avoid fatigue
B) To prevent injuries
C) To accommodate changing abilities
D) Both B and C